SAVVY ORGANIC SHOPPER'S GUIDE

HOW TO GET TOP QUALITY ORGANIC FOOD AT UP TO AN UNBELIEVABLE 70 % DISCOUNT

TANIA BELKIN

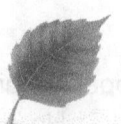

Copyright Notice

Copyright © 2013 Tania Belkin.

Published by Tania Belkin, All rights reserved.

All content contained within the "Savvy Organic Shopper's Guide" is copyright © of Tania Belkin. All literary work contained within the "Savvy Organic Shopper's Guide" belongs to and is the sole property of its respective author.

Reproduction, copying, or any other form of use of any part of the "Savvy Organic Shopper's Guide" is STRICTLY FORBIDDEN without express permission from the author. If perjury is discovered, the offenders will be prosecuted to the full extent of the law.

These rules have been established to protect the rights and ownership of the author and to ensure that her work is upheld as her own.

Library and Archives Canada Cataloguing in Publication:

Tania, Belkin

Savvy Organic Shopper's Guide: How to Get Top Quality Organic Food At Up To an Unbelievable 70 % Discount / Tania Belkin.

Health & Fitness. I. Title.

ISBN   978-0-9877845-2-0

DEDICATION

I dedicate this book to you, my reader. I hope this book sets you on a path towards a healthier life and more meaningful experiences.

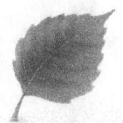

CONTENTS

	Acknowledgments	i
	Preface	1
	Introduction	5
1	Buying in Bulk	7
2	Co-op For Food & House Cleaning Products	13
3	Organic Farmers' Markets	18
4	Buying Straight From the Farm Itself	22
5	Distributors End-of-the-Month Sale	29
6	Proper Storage (Quick overview)	31
7	Resources vs. Resourcefulness	35
8	The Best Alternatives to Organic is Non-GMO	40
9	The Dirty Dozen with a Grain of Salt	43
10	Planning Ahead and Creating Your Buying Guide	47
11	Keep Looking	51
12	Where to Start	53
13	Never Shop When You are Hungry	55
14	No Matter What, Buy the Best Quality Food	57
15	Change Your Priorities	59
	Endnotes	62

ACKNOWLEDGMENTS

I would like to express my deepest gratitude to my husband Eddy, partner and editor whose loving support helped me see this project through to its completion.

To David and Jonathan my children, who gave me space to write and for giving me the pride and joy that only a parent can feel.

I owe a debt of gratitude to my editor and friend Marilyn Abramovitz, who challenged me to produce a better book.

Last but not least, I am so thankful to my friends who supported me and provided me with helpful feedback and camaraderie at all stages of this book.

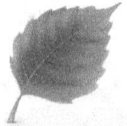

Preface

Why Eating Organic is Important

Organic food, whether produce or meat is grown and bred without antibiotics and synthetic chemicals such as: growth hormones, pesticides, insecticides and herbicides. Consumption of organic foods may reduce exposure to pesticide residues and antibiotic-resistant bacteria.[1] It also supports the humane treatment of animals being bred for meat or eggs. Organic food brings important benefits to our ecology [2], and to the future of agriculture.

Animals

Organic standards call for humane treatment of animals. Farmers are not allowed to put their animals in cages full-time. The animals must have a minimum required space to roam around. Farmers are not allowed to feed antibiotics and growth hormones to their livestock. In addition, organically-raised animals can only be fed organically ground crops that haven't been treated with synthetic herbicides and pesticides.[3]

Crops

Organic crop producers need to be follow strict protocols - no synthetic herbicides and pesticides, nothing that can be potentially harmful or damaging to animals and to the ecology. [3]

You are probably wondering how organic farmers control pests and weeds. There are many environmentally safe practices that have been used for centuries to achieve results in a natural way. These practices may not be as effective as using conventional industrial chemicals and they are also more labor intensive, but many environmentalists claim the benefits are well worth it.

Study after study has shown that organic farming practices are ecologically kinder. [2] Some studies now support the hypothesis that there is a link between the use of Organophosphate Pesticides and Attention-Deficit/Hyperactivity Disorder (ADHD) in children. [4]

While it is true that conventional foods only contain small residues of herbicides and pesticides, still, because we are exposed to so many environmental chemicals, these can be cumulatively damaging to our health. Therefore, if it is reasonably simple to eliminate some chemicals from our diet, I would rather do so and err on the side of caution. That's one of the primary reasons why I firmly believe that consuming organic food is more beneficial to our health than conventional food.

As far as nutritional value goes, there are studies that show organic food as having only a marginally better nutritional profile compared to conventional food. In the opinion of some researchers, the added expense doesn't warrant buying organic food.

To this I say better soil management, better quality soil, fewer environmental impacts makes for better food all around. Besides, if you buy organic food at a substantial savings, in my opinion, the balance swings clearly in favor buying organic food.

In addition, many maintain that organic food tastes better. Maybe it's because many organic growers harvest their produce when they are fully ripe, and use heirloom species known for their exceptional flavor. For example, I know of one farmer that cultivates over 40 varieties of heirloom tomatoes during one growing season.

If you want to know more about why eating organic is better, there are many resources to confer, below are a few you can start with:

http://www.sciencedaily.com/releases/2005/03/050

328182123.htm

http://www.generationsoforganic.org/health-nutrition/grains/

http://www.organic-center.org/science.events.php?action=view&report_id=148

Organic Food May Differ from Conventional

If you are new to organics you may notice that some food looks and feels different than the conventional food that you are used to.

For example, organic peanut butter may have oil separated and floating on top. This is because there are no binding agents to create a uniform texture. You just need to mix the nut butter after opening.

Also, since prepared organic food generally has fewer additives to enhance taste, at first taste, you may detect less flavor. However, as you begin your transition into organic food, you will soon educate your palette and realize that what you taste is actually very flavorful. You will begin to discriminate between the natural taste of food and all the additives you were previously accustomed to eating. Then you will appreciate the natural flavors of organic food.

Introduction

Yes, it is possible to save as much as 70% on your organic food bills!

The Savvy Organic Shopper's Guide explores different ways of buying organic food from various sources so that you can take advantage of great savings.

While savings are great, there are also many additional benefits to using the methods outlined in this guide:

You will be able to recognize and buy higher quality food.

You will be able to get fresher food.

You can be properly informed about where your food comes from, how it is grown and how it is made.

By reading this guide, you also will gain a better understanding of how to identify known and trusted sources of high quality foods. This will set your mind at ease and help eliminate nagging doubts about improper food handling, about cruelty to animals and about countries of origin that maintain lower standards, as well as environmental pollution. Making informed decisions about your food purchases is something from which we can all benefit.

Happy reading.

1

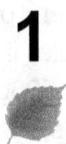

Buying in Bulk

Buying organic food in bulk is one of the most advantageous and easiest ways to start transitioning your family into consuming organic food, especially for products that have a long shelf life such as beans and legumes.

If you don't have a large family, you probably believe that this will not work for you. Not true. You can still benefit from buying food in bulk if you store it properly. For more information on food storage, please see chapter 6.

For a free food storage guide please see: http://proorganicliving.com/bonus

Why does buying organic food in bulk provide the most value for your dollar? Because the consumer price is often triple or quadruple when you buy your food in small quantities.

Having been in the Organic Food Business as a manufacturer and distributor for over 10 years, I am well aware of this principle. This is because smaller packaging adds enormous cost. Materials such as paper bags, labels and the boxes products are packaged in are not very pricey per unit, but costs do add up. For example, if you repackage a 10 kg bag of rice (bulk) into 500g bags, you would need 20 bags, instead of one, 19 additional labels, boxes for transportation plus extra labor. In addition you would incur some losses due to spillage during packaging. All these factors play into increasing your cost as a retail consumer.

Here's another example: consider buying sliced cheese versus block cheese. In many cases small packages of sliced cheese, e.g. 6 oz packages are equal in price to 1 lb. cheese blocks. The sliced cheese is hard to produce. This is because it is difficult to slice cheese without breaking some pieces. As a result, there is a lot of wastage. The broken slices need to be sold at a cheaper rate as a different product, e.g. grated cheese. Because the cheese manufacturer incurs a certain amount of loss, this translates into higher prices to the consumer. However, when you open a 1lb. block of cheese, you can keep this cheese refrigerated for weeks thus providing you with greater savings.

You may be thinking that block cheeses are less convenient. That's true, but you need to decide what is more important to you at the moment.

Savvy Organic Shopper's Guide

Convenience items usually cost more often much more. Also, many convenience items rarely provide the best quality because of the many food additives such as preservatives, artificial flavors and the use of lesser quality ingredients. (Cost saving measures.)

You may also be thinking that if I buy in bulk, I will eat more because I have more. If this is the case, then buy those foods that you want to consume more of - healthy foods such as vegetables and fruit, but not chocolates and candies.

Opting for bulk purchases helps manufacturers reduce their costs by about 50%. In addition, they are also happy to reduce their carbon footprint. Using less packaging, less paper and plastic, translates into using less energy which means less pollution. Minimal packaging also means that there are fewer things to dispose of and recycle. All this translates into a smaller carbon footprint.

Which Foods are Appropriate to Buy in Bulk?

- ➢ Organic Beans,
- ➢ Organic Legumes
- ➢ Organic Grains,
- ➢ Organic Pasta,
- ➢ Organic Flour,

- Organic Nuts,
- Organic Nut Butters,
- Organic Dried Fruits,
- Organic Coffee,
- Organic Tea,
- Organic Root vegetables,
- Organic Apples or any fruit that will keep well,
- Organic Frozen Meats and Poultry,
- Dairy products, especially those that freeze well like butter and cheese when it is grated,
- And anything you can think of that you will use before it goes bad.

Do You Care Where Your Food Comes From?

An additional advantage of buying bulk is that you can more easily determine the origin of the product. This is because bulk food often comes in large bags with the name of the farm or manufacturer stamped on it. The original manufacturing formats are often large. And, as I mentioned above, you may want to avoid organic food from suspicious sources because of environmental pollution, radiation, low hygiene standards and the like.

Always Compare Prices

But don't assume that buying large quantities always pays off. You still need to do price comparisons. It is very possible, and I have seen this myself, that grains or other commodities sold from dispensers in bulk are priced the same per ounce as items in individual packages. This is because there are costs associated with offering bulk: pest and bug control, lost shelf space, cost of the bags into which the grains are dispensed and waste by spillage. Also, some retailers exploit the consumers' belief that "more is cheaper" and charge the same price per unit as per smaller formats.

Pay Attention to Storage

The product's shelf life often depends on how it is stored. If you store your organic grains properly, they can last for years while improper storage will dramatically reduce their lifespan to as little as a few months. You must always start with high quality products. Proper storage does nothing to improve the quality of an inferior product.

Tania Belkin

Not all Bulk Packaged Food is Good

Do you really need to buy confectionary in bulk? My experience is that by doing so, you spend more. True, instead of the five dollars per chocolate bar you will have paid three dollars. However, instead of a once per week treat, you now eat three bars per week. So, rather than spending five dollars per week you end up spending nine dollars and you'll probably pack on a few unnecessary pounds on top of it.

Savings that result from buying in bulk are all good if you make use of all the food you purchase, or at least most of it. Throwing away part of your bulk purchases due to spoilage for example, is wasteful and not a good budgetary decision. Think it over before buying bulk. To help you better understand your needs; please see the 'Understanding Your Needs' section 10.

2

Co-op For Food & House Cleaning Products

What is a Co-op?

There are many different co-operatives and they all operate a bit differently but the main idea is the same. You pay a small fee to become a member; in return, you are able to purchase items you need at reduced prices. Some Co-ops may give members an opportunity to work there as volunteers. In exchange for services, volunteers will sometimes get even better prices. Co-op's are usually set up to help people live ecologically and socially responsible lives.

Essentially, a co-op is not owned by one person, but by all of its members. Its main purpose is to offer products at a fair price. Co-ops look for products that offer good value and try to work within the smallest profit-range possible. They work to balance fair price with covering their expenses, such as rent and employee salaries. Generally, their mandate is to make organic, ecological, fair trade and local products more accessible to people.[5]

Not all Co-ops are Created Equal

You may come across some co-ops that don't offer you a significant price advantage. Some may even ask for a large sum to become a member and or expect you to make a minimum monthly purchase. If their criterion sounds too complicated or too involved, I suggest looking elsewhere for a co-op that will not constrain you as much. Still, many co-ops do offer great savings to their members and it is definitely worth exploring this option.

House Cleaning Products

You will discover that many co-ops offer ecological and green house cleaning products. You can generally expect to pay much less for these eco-cleaners than at your local grocery store.

Savvy Organic Shopper's Guide

This is because co-ops buy these soaps and cleaners in bulk. They get the cleaners in large industrial-size containers and transfer them to dispensers, thus allowing consumers to fill their own bottles. Consumers can either bring their own empty bottles of shampoo, liquid soap; dishwasher and laundry detergents or they can buy new empty plastic bottles at the co-op and use those.

The underlying principle here is the same as buying food in bulk: Consumers benefit by reducing the resources manufacturers' need to create smaller packaging thus saving a great deal in the process.

Let me give you a quick example. I came to my local co-op with an empty shampoo bottle I previously purchased. I filled it up paying two dollars and change. Originally this bottle of shampoo cost me over ten dollars. Isn't that amazing? I got an 80% savings right off the bat.

Please note, not everything you buy will get you the same degree of savings. But, if you look around, you will be able to find many of your favorite household and personal products at a great discount.

One little inconvenience: You may need to pay a small fee to become a member. This could run in the neighborhood of $10 to $25 per year. But it's well worth it.

Food Co-ops

Food co-ops work by the same principle described above. Some co-ops offer both food and household products at the same location and may also carry personal care products, ecological household items as well as clothes.

Community

Good co-ops are there to serve the community. They support and promote local producers of ecological, fair trade and organic products. They look for ways to give back to their members in more ways than one.

For example, my local co-op schedules many free events throughout the year. These include fairs, lectures, information kiosks and workshops. It also promotes a 'buy nothing' day once a year during the busiest sales season. Consumers are invited to attend and are not expected to purchase anything. Its purpose is to show members that co-ops are not there just to make a buck. On this 'buy nothing' day, activities are provided for adults and children, as well as information kiosks. On Earth Day, they give away free native trees and bushes for planting.

Co-ops also help other likeminded people and businesses promote their products. They often allow producers of organic and eco-friendly products set up tables in their store to showcase their products and to inform co-op members and customers about their services.

The annual member's fee at the co-op I frequent is only ten dollars, and even this, is voluntary. By becoming a member you will have access to more discounts on pretty much anything at the store.

A good co-op listens to its members and tries to implement their suggestions; whether it's about the music they play in the store or about a new line of products they should look into.

Co-ops are there to encourage you to live a more ecologically- minded lifestyle. Many members will bring their plastic bags, plastic bottles and empty yogurt containers to be reused by other co-op customers.

If you find a good co-op, you will also start feeling a sense of belonging.

3

Organic Farmers' Markets

Generally speaking, purchasing foods directly from a farmer's market is a great idea.

Fresh, Fresh, Fresh

You will often find the healthiest and most vibrant looking vegetables at these farmers' markets. This is because these organic vegetables were either harvested a day before they came to market or even the very same morning! Can it get any fresher? The freshness of these products is unbeatable.

Price

Yes, the prices of produce found at these

farmers' markets, most of the time, are excellent. And they get even better as it gets later into the season when farmers are harvesting the last of their garden produce and want to sell the remaining harvest quickly. Thus, in late October you can buy a box of peppers for the price of a small basket or a bucket of apples for the price of a dozen apples.

Other Benefits of a Farmer's Market

Since most organic consumers are environmentally and fair-trade conscious, by supporting local organic farmers' markets they are also contributing towards bettering economic and environmental issues globally, like,

- ➢ Prevention of soil erosion,
- ➢ Preservation of soil fertility,
- ➢ Sustainable farming,
- ➢ The Economic welfare of local communities.

Generally, vegetables or any food grown on a small scale are better quality, more nutritious and produced in a more environmentally sound way. Long travel time has been shown to reduce the nutritional value of food and to have a negative impact on the environment. The fresher the food, the longer it will keep, thus reducing food waste. As well, small scale organic farmers take better care of the soil and the environment at large, as this is a requirement of organic agriculture. Simultaneously, by doing so, you are supporting your own community. How cool is that?

You'll Also Get to Meet the Farmer

This is a great place to meet farmers from who you may end up buying your food for years. Many farmers have their own delivery system: They will either deliver their products to your house or to a designated drop-off point where you can pick up your order during the winter months.

For farmers, a farmer's market is a good place to acquire new customers. And for you, as a consumer, these markets are great venues in which to find a farmer you can trust.

The second benefit - which I find priceless - is that you will know exactly where your food is coming from. And, should you have any concerns you have someone to turn to for answers. For example, a lot of organic food is grown in foreign countries with very questionable organic standards and this is a big concern for organic consumers. So, if you know the farmers and you feel you can trust them, this is a big advantage. Additionally, many farmers are open to having consumers visit their farms. By doing so, one gets additional confirmation as to whether one wants to buy food from him or not.

4

Buying Straight From the Farm Itself

Yet another easy way of getting organic food at rock bottom prices is going directly to the farmer.

Price, Price, Price

By going directly to the farm itself, you are saving the farmer time and money. Think about it, the farmer doesn't have to load his truck, drive for an hour or two to bring his produce to you and then drive back from the city. And, there are no fees for him to pay for a place at the market or at the drop-off point. Most farmers would rather stay at the farm and do what they love - farming.

All of the above make it so much more attractive for a farmer to give you the best possible price. If you buy some of your food in larger quantities you can get even better discounts. As an example, you can buy a big bag of potatoes or apples knowing they will keep for long time. This also applies to meat that can always be frozen. Why not ask if you can get a better price if you buy in larger quantities? However, always compare prices, no matter what.

Sometimes a farmer will charge you the same price whether you drive to their farm or if you meet him in town. Make sure you don't lose time because you think that you are getting significant savings, when in reality you aren't. Always ask whether you will get a better price by going to the farm and then make your decision.

I have done both. Most of the time, I have my order delivered. But, on occasion, I drive to the farm to get to know the farmer and see his operation. My children enjoy it too; they like visiting the farm and spending a day out of town. Eating berries straight from the bush or running with chickens in the open yard is always a great experience for them.

Do You Know Where Your Food is Coming From?

Bear in mind that buying from the farm is an excellent way of getting to know where your food is coming from. At the same time, you will also get to know the farmer and will observe first-hand his farming practices.

People are generally proud of what they do, and farmers are no exception. You will also learn a great deal about farming, in case you decide to plant your own garden one day.

What Can You Buy From a Farmer?

Depending where you live and what is grown in your particular area, some products can include:

- Meats,
- Poultry,
- Eggs,
- Cheese,
- Milk and dairy products,
- Bread and other baked goods,
- Vegetables,
- Fruits,
- Berries,
- Nuts,

- ➢ Seeds,
- ➢ dry fruits, dry mushrooms ...
- ➢ and anything else that is grown in your area.

Note: you can freeze or process many of the above and they will last you throughout the winter and beyond. Doing so allows me, for example, to make fresh (five- minute) blueberry jams for my children all winter long. They love my warm fresh berry jam on a cold school morning.

Volunteering at the Farm

Some farmers have programs set up for volunteers. This can be of benefit to you and your family. I know one local organic farmer who accepts as much time and effort as you are willing to give.

Why Should You Volunteer?

Get Your Food for Free

OK, maybe not completely free, you may pay something depending on how much food you need but, if you do pay, it will be less than if you bought the food outright.

Helping and Giving

There is an old axiom: Who gains more, the giver or the receiver? And the answer is - the giver.

Giving to others are the two biggest gifts we can give ourselves. It helps us feel worthy. And, if you get your children to lend a helping hand, you will very likely see an almost immediate change in them. You will see pride in their eyes.

Bringing Your Family to the Farm

By going to a farm your children will learn a great deal and get to appreciate their food more. They will also experience the symbiotic relationship between giving and receiving.

Additionally, they will begin to understand the food- growing cycle.

They will appreciate farmers, and understand how hard they work to produce the food we often take for granted. In the long run, by volunteering, children become more appreciative, more caring and more grateful.

I Am a City Person, What Can I Do at the Farm?

Anything you like. You can tie up their flowers, fix the fence harvest vegetables, sort through the harvested berries, and so on. You get the idea. Many 'jobs' at the farm are lots of fun.

Reciprocal Relationship

When you volunteer at the farm you get to know the farmer more personally and will probably develop a better relationship with him. Doing so can pay dividends for years to come.

For example, when the farmer has one dozen of eggs left and three people want these eggs, who do you think gets it? Is it the person who rolled up his sleeve and helped out? Or, is it someone who just gives his order, receives his food and never calls until he needs something again?

You guessed it. If you help just a bit, people appreciate and remember this. In return, you will get all kinds of favors - the kind that you never thought possible.

All things being equal, people would rather do business with people they like. All things not being equal, people still would rather do business with people they like.[6]

As well, if you ever want to grow your own garden, you will have gotten yourself a free mentor. You will get plenty of tried and true free advice - practical tips and tricks that often take years to learn. You will learn what works in *your* zone, not just what a book tell you will grow. Over the years, many of my flower beds failed because I relied exclusively on what gardening books recommended. Advice from books doesn't always work, whereas advice from my farmer always works.

5

Distributors End-of-the-Month Sale

Some food distributors designate one day per month to selling selected merchandise directly to the consumer. This usually takes place on the weekend, for instance, every last Saturday of the month. If you are fortunate to have such a distributor in your district, you can save a bundle of money.

What Do They Sell?

They sell damaged packages or food that will expire within the next six months or so. The store may need to have a six to twelve- month shelf life to guarantee the sale of the product. You, as a consumer may be fine with a two to three month shelf life before the food expires – that is, as long as you don't buy more than you need. Remember to always check the expiry date on any packaging.

'Damaged' packages tend to be of little real significance: The packages usually have a small defect. For instance, a cereal box can have a bent corner, a scratch on the package or a defective label. The food is perfectly fine; it's just that the package just doesn't look good on a shelf. Shipping it back to manufacturer may cost more than it's worth.

What Will You Save

You will often save 50 - 70%. Sometimes more. You are not going to get all of your food this way, just some. But this can significantly add to your overall savings. These are usually sold on a cash-and-carry basis.

6

Proper Storage (Quick overview)

Your food will last longer - a lot longer - if you store it properly.

To get a full version of my food storage guide go to http://proorganicliving.com/bonus.

Here is a quick overview:

Berries

Berries are an excellent source of vitamins and a fabulous treat in the winter. They freeze well and keep for several years when properly stored.

Buy your berries, such as blueberries, strawberries, raspberries and cranberries, in season. It's a good idea to buy them in bulk to secure additional savings. Wash or rinse your berries through a sieve and then dry them. If your berries came in small containers, you can use those for storage, but rinse the containers out well before reusing. Then put your berries back in their original containers. Place the containers in individual or larger zip-lock bags and directly into the freezer. If you don't have containers, zip-lock bags will do just fine.

Leafy Vegetables

Lettuce, spinach and other salad leaves, celery & leafy vegetables such as Bok Choy and Kale will keep well if properly packaged. Always keep them refrigerated. Put bunches of them into a plastic bag and loosely tie them. Leave some room for the leaves to breath. If these leaves are wet, or slightly moist, wrap them in paper towels before placing them into plastic bags. Also, don't pack these bags too tightly. And don't place anything on top of the bags. If you get your salad fresh and in good condition, salad will keep for a month or more.

Frozen Fish, Poultry and Meat

When freezing your meats, poultry and fish, there is a significant principle involved when it comes to their packaging: The less air exposure, the longer your food will keep. Vacuum sealing is very useful, especially as regards meat. Also, the quality of your frozen food largely depends on the type of freezer you own and where in the freezer your food is placed.

Chest freezers are better if your want to keep your food for long-term storage. Especially if the food is placed at the bottom of the freezer and is covered or placed in a box with airtight packaging. This way, it will keep the longest. If you place your food in the freezer door, which you open often and if the packaging is not airtight, then you can only expect your food to last several weeks at best.

Seeds and Nuts

To preserve freshness, shelled nuts and seeds are best kept refrigerated, or in a cool, dry place. Nuts that are in the shell have a longer shelf life. If you store them cool and dry, they will keep for one to two years. Roasting your nuts may also help to prolong shelf-life, but will decrease their nutritional value.

Bran, Oatmeal and Flakes

For short-term storage bran and flakes are fine at room temperature. If you are planning to keep them longer than a few months, or if you live in a hot climate, you will be well advised to refrigerate them.

Again, place them either in tightly sealed jars or in sealed plastic bags.

To obtain my complete guide free, go to: http://proorganicliving.com/bonus/

7

Resources vs. Resourcefulness

When one lacks resources – for instance, either time, money, household help - resourcefulness can kick in to compensate.[7]

Make Your Own Food

I know many people, myself included, who spend much time preparing food at home using the best-quality ingredients. More time spent at home preparing food, usually results in less time eating out. This saves you a bundle, as well. You will then be in the better position to afford to buy more organic food: Buying prepared foods, whether organic or not, adds considerably to the bottom line.

In my family, we bake our own breads. Doing so takes very little time. It costs pennies to make beautiful organic bread at home compared to the store-bought ones. Nothing compares to a fresh bread right out of the oven. I know what ingredients we used and how it was handled. This is important to me since I tend to be somewhat of a hygiene freak.

We make our own jams from our frozen berries our own sauerkraut, kefir, cottage cheese, kombucha tea and more. We're not the only ones. We have friends who make all their breads and pastries, jams, tomato sauce, pickles, yogurt, natto, mustards, just to name a few.

I'm not suggesting that you need to make all your food yourself, just pick a few items you think you will enjoy making and you will find the effort very gratifying.

Grow Some of Your Own Vegetables

If you enjoy planting flowers, you may enjoy planting a vegetable garden as well. You can buy sprouted plants. Or you can grow your vegetable plants from seed.

People who like gardening reap many benefits:

- They get in contact with the soil,
- They get sunshine and fresh air,
- They get to spend time enjoying nature,
- They get to reap the rewards of their labor,
- They learn self-reliance and sustainability,
- The save on their food bills.

If you are not in-love with the idea of gardening or believe that you don't have a green thumb, I understand. But, if you are open to it, think of how you can easily transform seeds that cost pennies or plants that cost two or three dollars into top quality organic food that costs a fortune in the store. And, by the way, a green thumb can always be developed. Actually most of the work is done by the plants and not by you! And you can potentially reap ten to twenty dollars worth of produce per plant.

Other Ways to Reduce Your Food Costs

Find Alternatives to Bottled Water

When you filter your own water or distil it, you will immediately see the savings. By using bottled water, you are not only wasting a lot of money but are also facing increased health risks. There many studies that found bacteria in bottled water. [8] Plastic bottles also tend to leach unhealthy chemicals into your water. [9]

Start by getting a simple water filter that will remove fluoride and chlorine as well as other particulate matter from your water.

When leaving your house, remember to take the water with you in a stainless steel canteen. Just make sure that your bottle is real stainless steel, not aluminum on the inside; or worse yet, aluminum coated with a thin plastic layer.

Eliminate Convenience Items

Convenience items are those foods that are ready to eat. They are usually sold in small packages and cost multiples times more than what they should. True, using them saves us time, but we are paying big bucks for that convenience.

These can include:

- ➤ A five dollar cup of coffee,
- ➤ A cookie or muffin to go with your coffee,
- ➤ Ready to eat soups in a cup - just add hot water,
- ➤ Bottled water - small format,
- ➤ Vending machine sandwiches,
- ➤ And many, many others.

8

The Best Alternatives to Organic is Non-GMO

What would be a second best option, when organic food is not accessible?

When we don't have access to organic food, food labeled as 'Natural' quickly comes to mind. But as you may know, 'natural' is a vague term that has been exploited by clever marketing. Additionally, by reading the ingredients you will often discover that there is nothing "natural" about many products labeled 'Natural'. That is why, the second best alternative to 'organic' is 'GMO- free' products.

What are GMOs?

'GMO' stands for genetically modified organisms. These are organisms that have been biotechnologically created by splicing and combining genes sometimes from different species. Doing this creates more resilient plants. But, how safe it is for human consumption? The jury is still out, but, growing evidence is pointing more to health risks rather than to benefits. [10]

Although it would be nearly impossible to say that your food is 100% GMO- free, you can realistically come pretty close to obtaining that.

What are the Products Contaminated by GMOs?

When we hear the term 'GMO', many of us automatically think grains and produce such as: soy, corn, canola and vegetables. But, if we closely examine our milk, meat, poultry, eggs and honey, to mention just a few, we come to realize how these products can be highly contaminated by GMOs, as well. This is because there is a high risk of GMOs in animal feed.

How Can We Protect Ourselves from GMOs?

The Non-GMO Project resource identifies those products that contain near-zero GMOs. The Non-GMO Project is a non-profit organization that offers non-GMO labeling to participating food producers. It uses third party verification. This helps participating producers follow the best practices for avoiding GMO contaminated products.

To find out more about this organization, please visit the Non-GMO Project at http://www.nongmoproject.org. There you will find a list of participating producers as well as products which are non-GMO compliant.

9

The Dirty Dozen with a Grain of Salt

If, for some reason, you can't buy all your food organic, then there is always the dirty dozen and clean fifteen list to which you should refer. The dirty dozen is a list of fruits and vegetables that are the most heavily sprayed with chemicals such as herbicides and pesticides while the clean fifteen is a list of vegetables and fruits that are least sprayed. Unfortunately, the later list is not as clean as suggested. For example, sweet corn is on the clean 15 list, but while it is probably true that corn is sprayed much less than apples, it may nonetheless be genetically modified as well as sprayed with 'Roundup', which has been deemed very harmful to humans and the ecology. Roundup is a synthetic herbicide used to eliminate weeds. [11] Virtually all non-organic corn is genetically modified. That is one of the reasons corn syrup has been getting such bad press.

The Dirty Dozen:

- Apples,
- Celery,
- Sweet Bell Peppers,
- Peaches,
- Strawberries,
- Nectarines (imported),
- Grapes,
- Spinach,
- Lettuce,
- Cucumbers,
- Blueberries (domestic),
- Potatoes,

Plus:

- Green Beans,
- Kale/Collard Greens.

The Clean 15:

- Onions,
- Sweet corn,
- Pineapples,
- Avocados,
- Cabbage,
- Sweet Peas,
- Asparagus,
- Mangoes,
- Eggplant,
- Kiwi,
- Cantaloupe (domestic),
- Sweet Potatoes,
- Grapefruit,
- Watermelon,
- Mushrooms.

While it is probably safe to use most of the foods listed as "Clean" – there are some I suspect that may not be as "clean" as presumed. As mentioned above, to my knowledge, most non-organic corn is genetically modified. I have also seen several negative reports about watermelon, kiwi and other fruit grown in China. [12]

10

Planning Ahead and Creating Your Buying Guide

The saying goes: If you fail to properly plan, you are planning to fail. It's much easier to buy organic food on a budget if you plan ahead. Weekly planning is the easiest to manage. You know what your family likes to eat and in what quantities. It's fast and easy to plan a menu and shopping list. Those who are serious about what they eat, plan ahead.

On the other hand, if you buy all of your groceries at the last minute, just as you need them, you are probably paying a premium and likely sacrificing quality for convenience.

Plan Ahead

You can also plan your winter needs during the

summer and fall. If you have a room that is cool, you can buy apples and root vegetables in the fall, when they are cheap, and store them for a couple of months. I know people who are very busy in the fall buying their food for the winter.

Vegetables like potatoes, beets, carrots and squash keep for many months. Late fall apples are usually excellent keepers as well.

I buy beautiful butternut squash from a farmer friend. We eat them all fall, winter and spring, up until April or May.

Some people make their own pickled cucumbers, pickled tomatoes, tomato sauce and sauerkraut to last them throughout the winter.

Berries are in abundance and very inexpensive in the summer. Buy a case or two and store them in the freezer and you will appreciate your berry stash during the winter. To download a free guide on how to store food properly, please go to http://proorganicliving.com/bonus/

At home, we make use of our berries all winter long. We make a five-minute breakfast jam, bake with them and eat them slightly defrosted as a desert. My children love to put frozen berries in their teas to cool them down and add a burst of flavor on a cold school morning.

Again, remember - never buy more than you need. Just because the price is great, it's not free and there is no need to be wasteful.

Understand Your Needs

The basic rule is: If you don't regularly use very much of a particular product, don't buy it in large quantities. It will either go bad or you will get tired of it eventually. In the case of organic junk foods like chips, candies, etc., you will probably end up eating more of them than you should.

But, those foods your family consumes on a regular basis like rice or potatoes – it is easy to estimate how quickly a bag is consumed before it goes bad.

Understand Your Storage Capacity

If the food requires special storage like a cool place, refrigeration or freezing, think ahead and determine if you have enough room to store it.

On the other hand, if you have family or good friends with whom you buy in bulk have lots of space, you may ask them to store some of your food for you.

Understanding Shelf Life

Some foods have a short shelf life and need special attention. Always check the expiry dates.

Other foods have a longer shelf life, but by storing them improperly, you could shorten their shelf life by up to 75% or more. Therefore, you are always better off knowing how to properly store these foods before buying them.

11

Keep Looking

Prices change, people-in-charge change, margins on the product change. Periodically keep comparing prices and look for new sources. You may have to change your buying habits from time to time to get a bigger bang for your buck.

The 80/20 Rule

Can you get 100% of your organic food at the discounted prices? Probably not. But with a bit of work, you could likely get it at a discount 80% of the time and still realize significant savings.

We similarly apply this 80/20 rule to what our children eat. Ideally, we want them to eat organic food all the time. But I know this is not always possible. They will eat at their friends' houses, they will eat an occasional cupcake in school and they will get their grandmother to buy them junk food. I don't like it, but it happens sometimes so I don't complain. And as my children get older and more knowledgeable, they eat less and less junk foods.

12

Where to Start

Here are a few ways to start. Use whatever method works best for you.

Start by Replacing the 'Most Polluted' Foods With Organic Foods.

The most polluted foods are those that contain the greatest amount of harmful substances, for example: dairy products meats, poultry and eggs. [13]

The reason this is so is because of suspected antibiotics and growth hormones in their feed. In addition, animals also eat grains that are heavily sprayed with pesticides, herbicides and are, possibly, genetically modified as well.

Residues of all these substances end up on your dinner plate. This is not the most appetizing thought, is it?

Start with What Your Eat the Most

My family, for example, eats an incredible amount of fruits and vegetables. So, it is important for us to find a farmer's market where we are able for get most of our organic fruits and vegetables at reasonable prices.

Also, seek out those foods that are readily available, so you can find them with little or no effort.

If you have an organic market near you, start with that.

If you know an organic farmer, ask him if you can visit his farm.

If you know a store nearby that sells organic food in bulk, pay them a visit.

13

Never Shop When You are Hungry

You have heard this advice before, but now it is officially proven and backed up by research. [14]

When you shop on an empty stomach you are much more likely to buy higher calorie foods like junk foods and you are also extremely likely to spend more money. This is because when you are hungry, your brain increasingly looks for a reward such as, high calorie foods.

The solution to this problem is simple: eat a healthy snack before you leave home. As you become saturated by your snack, your stomach will send a signal to your brain - 'famine is over'. You won't have this deep subconscious urge to 'fatten up'.

I would also suggest not bringing your young children shopping with you. My own experience, now supported by research, has taught me that we tend to spend more money and buy less healthy foods when we shop with our children. [15]

Making a list before going shopping is helpful, but it won't eliminate a few high-fat impulse purchases.

14

No Matter What, Buy the Best Quality Food

Fresh, organic, top quality food should be a priority for everyone, not to just an elite few. Your food affects your moods, your energy level and the clarity of your thinking. The food you eat makes a big difference in your overall health, in the quality of your life, on how you feel and on your longevity.

The purpose of this guide is to find a creative way of cutting your organic food costs without compromising the quality of your food.

By now you probably know that there are hidden costs in low quality food. It damages your health, the environment, and it will cost you more in medical bills and/or in elevated taxpayer dollars to cover the medical costs. This is in addition to the actual suffering and pain that people endure. When all is said and done, organic foods are by far less expensive in the long run than industrially-produced foods.

15

Change Your Priorities

You can learn to priorities your time and money.

Time

Sitting in front of the TV or computer screen at home, is not the best use of your time. Instead, put on your favorite music or motivational lecture and head to the kitchen to make a homemade healthy meal for your family. Doing this could be quite relaxing and meditative. Make it a priority and rearrange your daily routine.

Money

If something is important to you, you'll find a way to get it. The car you drive; the clothes you wear and those new electronic gadgets shouldn't be higher on your priority list than the foods you eat. Food is for you, other acquisitions like cars, designer clothes and gadgets are primarily there to impress people – some of who you may not even like.

Think about what you must buy and what can be avoided. Junk foods and convenience foods can easily be substituted for healthier snacks made at home. This would allot more money towards buying more organic foods and buying healthy ingredients in bulk.

Will this Take More Effort?

Perhaps in the beginning it will take more time and effort. But later on you will realize that you spend far less time in grocery stores and more time at home with your family. You can easily avoid or minimize the dreaded shopping trips with the kids. Mom, can I get that? Dad, can we buy that? I am hungry, let's stop at the store for snacks.... and on and on it goes. You know the drill.

They say exercise will add years to your life; proper food will add life to your years. Why, then, shouldn't we be enjoying our lives more fully?

Endnotes

Preface

Why Eating Organic is Important

[1] Annals of Internal Medicine: http://annals.org/article.aspx?articleid=1355685

[2] http://www.organic-center.org/science.events.php?action=view&report_id=148

[3] Government of Canada: Organic Production Systems General Principles and Management Standards 2011. The terms of the US-Canada equivalency agreement on organic production can be found on CFIA website.

[4] http://pediatrics.aappublications.org/content/early/2010/05/17/peds.2009-3058.abstract

Savvy Organic Shopper's Guide

Co-op For Food & House Cleaning Products

What is a Co-op

[5] *Wikapedia.com*, "Fair trade is an organized social movement that aims to help producers in developing countries achieve better trading conditions and promote sustainability. It advocates the payment of fair prices (higher prices) to exporters and raise higher social and environmental standards." http://en.wikipedia.org/wiki/Fairtrade (accessed September 22 2013)

Buying Straight From the Farmer

Reciprocal Relationship

[6] Quote from Jeffrey Gitomer.

Resources vs. Resourcefulness

[7] Quote from Tony Robbins.

Find Alternatives to Bottled Water

[8] http://www.ctvnews.ca/high-bacteria-levels-found-in-bottled-water-in-canada-1.515742 (accessed September 24 2013)

[9] http://www.dailymail.co.uk/health/article-2157423/Poisoned-plastic-Chemicals-water-bottles-food-packaging-linked-infertility-birth-defects-Scaremongering-truth.html (accessed September 24 2013)

The Best Alternatives to Organic is Non-GMO

What are GMOs?

[10] http://www.thegrocer.co.uk/topics/technology-and-supply-chain/monsanto-weedkiller-and-gm-maize-in-shocking-cancer-study/232603.article (accessed September 24 2013)

[10] http://www.dailymail.co.uk/sciencetech/article-2205509/Cancer-row-GM-foods-French-study-claims-did-THIS-rats--cause-organ-damage-early-death-humans.html?openGraphAuthor=%2Fhome%2Fsearch.html%3Fs%3D%26authornamef%3DSean%2BPoulter (accessed September 24 2013)

The Dirty Dozen with a Grain of Salt

[11] http://www.reuters.com/article/2013/04/25/roundup-health-study-idUSL2N0DC22F20130425 (accessed September 24 2013)

[12] http://www.cbsnews.com/2100-202_162-

20063538.html (accessed October 02 2013)

Where to Start

Start by Replacing the 'Most Polluted' Foods

[13] http://www.ewg.org/meateatersguide/a-meat-eaters-guide-to-climate-change-health-what-you-eat-matters/other-meat-concerns-antibiotics-hormones-and-toxins/ (accessed September 24 2013)

Never Shop When You are Hungry

[14]http://archinte.jamanetwork.com/article.aspx?articleid=1685889 (accessed September 24 2013)

[15] http://www.today.com/id/41259243/ns/today-money/t/supermarkets-wage-war-your-dollars/#.UkHXND-E5bV (accessed September 24 2013)
http://www.kitco.com?onepasswdfill=29A06EE2C4974E919EE34DD4FE5D06D0

www.ingramcontent.com/pod-product-compliance
Lightning Source LLC
LaVergne TN
LVHW051511070426
835507LV00022B/3055